Yoga

For Runners

Monique Joiner Siedlak

OSHUN
PUBLICATIONS

Printed in the United States of America

Second Edition 2018

ISBN-13: 978-1-948834-40-7

Publisher
www.oshunpublications.com

Disclaimer
All the material contained in this book is provided for educational and informational purposes only. No responsibility can be taken for any results or outcomes resulting from the use of this material. While every attempt has been made to provide information that is both accurate and effective, the author does not assume any responsibility for the accuracy or use/misuse of this information.

Yoga Poses Photos

Pixabay.com

Freepik.com

Dreamstime.com

Cover Design by Monique Joiner Siedlak

Cover Image by Pixabay.com

Logo Design by Monique Joiner Siedlak

Logo Image by Pixabay.com

Sign up to email list: www.mojosiedlak.com

Other Books in the Series

Yoga for Beginners

Yoga for Stress

Yoga for Back Pain

Yoga for Weight Loss

Yoga for Flexibility

Yoga for Advanced Beginners

Yoga for Fitness

Yoga for Energy

Yoga for Your Sex Life

Yoga: To Beat Depression and Anxiety

Yoga for Menstruation

Table of Contents

Introduction

Yoga is a form of exercise that focuses solely on body movement and position therefor the outcomes, the 'gains' aren't as important to a person performing yoga.

You are far more aware of your body while performing yoga. You can therefore gauge the effect an exercise is having on it. Your body is far more flexible and many runners cite Yoga as a solution for greater movement.

Anyone who is a runner will be surprised at how easily their legs give in when performing it. When running, you're only really targeting one certain area while others remain ignored. Yoga engages your muscles on all planes so it increases endurance.

Running is a purely physical exercise and of course, some might use it as a mental break, there really isn't a comparison to the workout your mind gets when you're working out. Yoga uses all muscle groups, your legs, toes, the back muscles your abdomen and the most important muscle of all, your brain!

One of the most important aspects to both forms of exercise is worked on and perfected. This is the act of breathing. Yoga IS the exercise of maintain your breathing and balancing it with your poses. If you're not breathing correctly during yoga, you might as well not even do the poses. Yoga builds the discipline of breathing. And if you're a runner, you KNOW the importance of maintain a correct breathing pattern. Honing that skill from yoga just might do the trick!

Standing Wide Legged Forward Fold Pose (Prasarita Padottanasana)

The Standing Wide Legged Forward Fold is a relaxing forward bend that stretches your hamstrings and back. This pose is from time to time also called the Wide-Legged Forward Bend the Standing Straddle, and, the Straddle Fold.

How to Do

Move your feet apart into a wide straddle. Your feet should be somewhat turned in so that the outside of your feet remain parallel. Start to develop into a forward bend, making sure that your effort is begun by the rotation of your pelvis forward. What you do not do all your forward bending with your spine. Keep a flat back as you move forward. Bringing your hands completely below your shoulders at first, start to walk your hands back, getting your wrists aligned with your ankles, if at all possible. Bend your elbows as you would with the Four-Limbed Staff Pose. You can furthermore make an effort by taking each of your big toes in a yogi toe lock with the parallel hand. You can pull slightly on your toes to increase your forward bend. A different option is to walk your hands back behind your ankles at the same time as you keep your arms straight. Try bringing your body weight onward into the balls of your feet to keep your hips in the same plane as your ankles. Engage your quadriceps and draw them upwards. Remain here for five to ten breaths, lengthening your spine on your inhalations and deepening your forward bend on your exhalations. To come out of the pose, bring your hands onto your hips and hold your back straight as you move up to stand.

Benefits

The Standing Wide Legged Forward Fold stretches your groin, hamstrings, and hips while decompressing your spine. Settles down the mind, reduces fatigue, mild depression, and apprehension.

Tips

If your head can with no trouble touch the floor, try narrowing your posture for a deeper hamstring stretch. If your head is on the floor, you may perhaps want to rise into a tripod headstand. Use blocks beneath your hands if they don't touch to the floor.

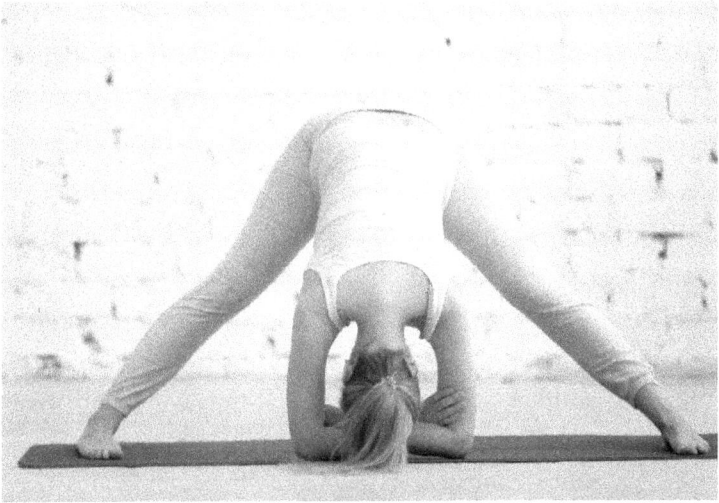

Standing Forward Fold Pose (Uttanasana)

Standing Forward Fold Pose is an important component of the Sun Salutations. This pose is used to train the body for deeper forward bends.

How to Do

Begin by Standing with your feet together. Bend your knees somewhat and bend your torso, not the lower back, over your legs, shift from your hips. Put your hands on the floor in front of you or next to your feet.

Breathe in and expand your chest to elongate your spine. Keep your focus fixed forward.

Breathe out and press both legs straight. Raise your kneecaps and twist your upper and inner thighs back. Without hyperextending, maintain your legs straight.

Extend your torso down without rounding your back, on an exhalation. Stay long through your neck, lengthening the top of your head toward the ground. Pull your shoulders down your back.

Benefits

The Standing Forward Fold pose extends your spinal column and stretches the back muscles as well as the backs of your legs.

Tip

Bend your knees to increase the stretch in the backs of your legs. Take care not to straighten the knees by locking them back; as an alternative, allow them to straighten as the two ends of each leg move farther spaced out.

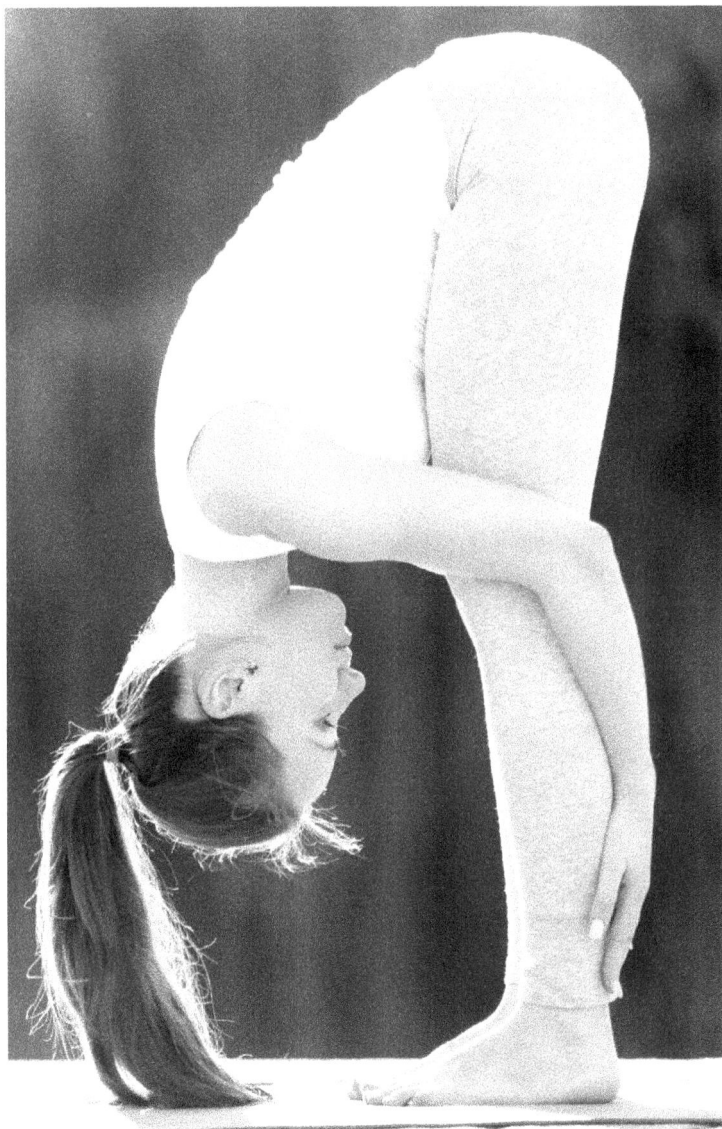

Pyramid Pose (Parsvottanasana)

The Pyramid Pose is a standing yoga posture that blends the advantages of balancing, forward bending and backward bending.

How to Do

With right foot forward From High Lunge Pose, move the back leg forward as much as necessary to straighten both legs. With the toes facing forward, keep the back foot flat on the floor. Round your spine moving your forehead towards the right knee, push into the heels and press the back of the knees in the direction of the back wall. Breathe and hold for four to ten breaths.

To release this pose, either breathe in the arms out and up with both legs straight or step the left foot back and bend the right knee into a lunge. Copy on the opposite side.

Benefits

The Pyramid Pose Builds up and tones the abdomen. It also Strengthens and stretches your entire leg and back.

Tip

When you forward bend, if your hands don't reach the floor, use blocks under them for support. It's important that your hands rest upon something other than your shin. Your feet should be parallel, not in line.

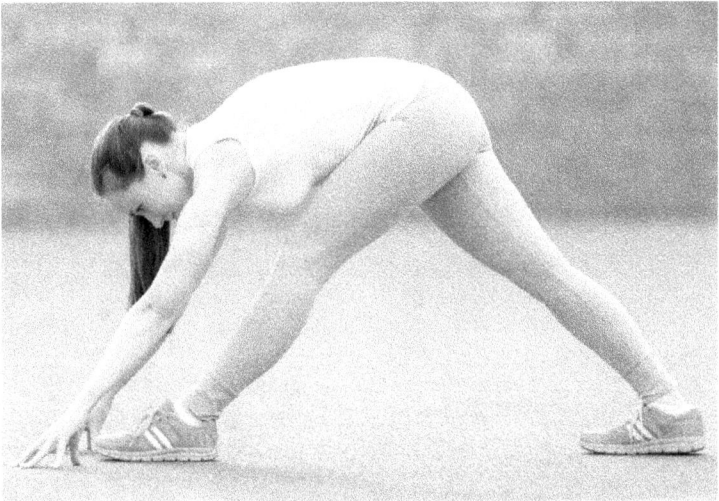

Triangle Pose (Utthita Trikonasana)

The Triangle Pose is a standing yoga pose that tones the legs, improves stability and diminishes stress.

How to Do

Start in the Mountain Pose. On an exhaling, step your right foot backward about three to four feet putting it parallel to the backside of your mat.

Angle your right foot in somewhat roughly fifteen to degrees, and line up the heel of your right foot with the heel of your left foot. Applying straight legs, firm your thighs without gripping into your knees, and bore the edge of your right big toe into your mat to begin and lift the arch of your front foot.

With an inhalation, spread your arms to shoulder height beside your body, parallel to the floor. Grasp out actively through the fingertips of both hands, palms facing down, and soften the tops of your shoulders.

Enter by extending your right hand forward and pivot at your right hip to bring your right hand down, having your front body and pelvis facing toward the left edge of your mat. Place your right hand on a block just outside the pinky toe edge of your right foot, if you have one. Place your right hand lightly on your right shin for support if a block isn't available.

Stretch your left arm straight up in the direction of the ceiling, firming your shoulder blades onto your back and widening the length from your middle fingertip on one arm to middle fingertip on the other arm when both arms are held out straight at your sides.

Lengthen evenly through both sides of your torso, and press into the support under your right hand to grow taller through your left fingertips and broaden across your collarbones.

Root down evenly through the four corners of both feet, paying particular attention to the outer edge of your back foot, which has a tendency to collapse inwards.

Keep your head in a neutral position or send your gaze up toward your left hand if it feels comfortable for your neck.

Stay in the pose for three to five full breaths. On an inhalation, send your look down and press firmly into the soles of both feet to bring yourself back vertical to stand, and step forward to the top of your mat. Reverse your feet and repeat on the other side.

Benefits

Opens your chest, shoulders and strengthens your legs, extends your groin, hamstrings, and hips.

Tips

If you feel unbalanced in the pose, support the back of your torso or your back heel against a wall.

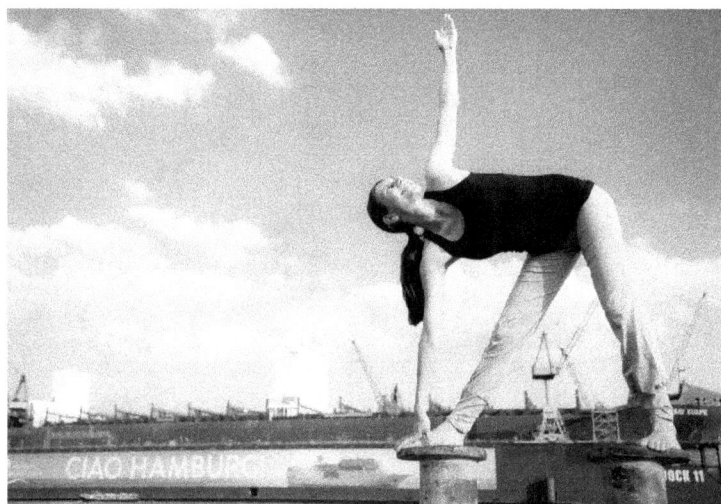

Head-To-Knee Forward Bend Pose (Janu Sirsasana)

The Head-to-Knee Forward Bend Pose is a deep, forward bend that soothes the mind and releases stress. It is frequently practiced near the end of a sequence, when the body is warm, to set up the body for even deeper forward bends.

How to Do

Start in a seated pose with your legs stretched. Bend the right leg, pulling the bottom of the foot to the upper inside of the right thigh. The right knee must rest steadily on the floor. Take both hands to both sides of the left leg. Breathe in and turn towards your extended leg. Breathe out and fold forward. Exhale slowly and deeply for three to five breaths. To come out of the pose, breathe in back to the beginning position. Repeat the other side.

Benefits

Helps tone your legs and burn the fats in your abdominal.

Tip

You can sit up on a blanket if your hips are tight. Place a strap about the extended foot, If you like or hold an end of the strap in each hand as you forward bend.

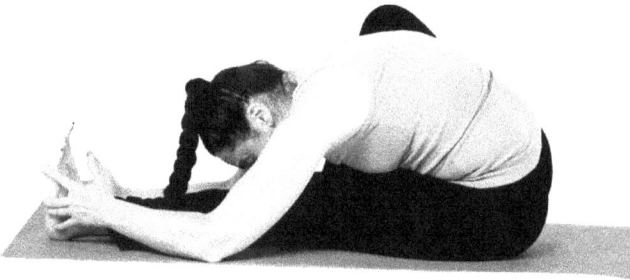

Eye of the Needle Pose (Sucirandhrasana)

The Eye of the Needle is a lying-down yoga pose that gets rid of rigidity in the outer hips and lower back. If you pass a great deal of time sitting, those muscles grow tight and short as a result of the lack of use.

How to Do

Start by reclining on your back with your knees bent and the bottom of your feet on the floor. Clasp your right knee into your chest. Cross the right ankle over your body and place it on the left thigh. Let the right knee relax away from your chest.

Raise your left foot off the floor and thread your right hand through your legs, which creates the eye of the needle, so that your hands come together on the back side of your left thigh. You can also, hold your hands on the front side of your left shin. Using your hands, pull your left thigh toward your chest. This will trigger your right hip to open. Keep both of your feet stretched. Breathe deeply and relax the right knee to open the hips.

Repeat on the other side.

Benefits

The Eye of the Needle stretches lower back opens hips reduces back pain.

Tip

The more you push your knee back, the more your hips will open and the deeper the stretch will be down the legs. If it feels painful because the stretch is too deep, angle your knee in the direction of your upper body. Use a yoga strap, tie or scarf by circling it around the back of the thigh and gripping each end with one hand, if you are unable to clasp your hands around your thigh.

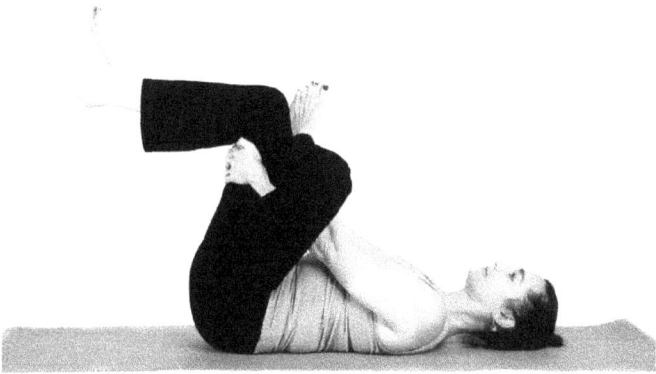

Half Lord of Fishes Pose (Ardha Matsyendrasana)

The Half Lord of Fishes Pose is a moderate to intense twist that encourages length of your spine, a base stretch for your outer hips, and brings forth growth through the chest and shoulders.

How to Do

Begin in a seated position with your legs straight in front of you. Bring in your knees up and bend them with the purpose of your feet are now flat on the floor. This is your beginning position. Bring your right leg beneath your left leg. Maintain your left leg in the starting position. Your right leg should bend at the knee and then keep close to your hip.

Taking your left leg, cross it over the left knee. Set your left foot flat on the floor on the outside of your right knee. Bring your right arm and reach up. Next slowly bend your arm at the elbow and place your elbow on your left knee. Take your left arm and place behind your back and use for a base.

Breathe in and out while either turning your head opposite to the way your back is stretching, or you can turn your head with your back.

Benefits

The Half Lord of Fishes Pose can restore and improve spinal range of motion. It also beneficial for backaches.

Tips

Maintain your right leg extended if you cannot steadily tuck it beneath your left buttock. Squeeze the left knee with your right arm if that feels better than bringing the right elbow outside the left knee. If you normally use a blanket or other prop under your sit bones for seated poses, it's fine to do that here as well.

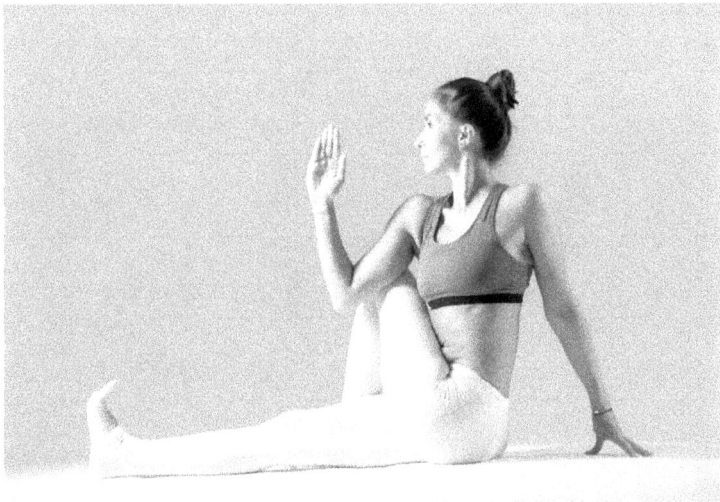

Butterfly Pose (Baddha Konasana)

The Butterfly Pose is a seated pose that strengthens and opens your hips and groin while decreasing abdominal pain.

How to Do

Sit with your knees near to your chest. Relax your knees out to each side and slightly press the bottoms of your feet together. Hold on to your ankles or feet.

Benefits

The Butterfly Pose is a good stretch for your inner thighs, groins, and knees. It helps improve the flexibility in your groin and hip area. When standing and walking for long hours, it removes fatigue.

Can give assistance from menstrual discomfort and menopause symptoms and smooth delivery if it's practiced on a regular basis until late pregnancy. Also helps in intestine and bowel movement.

Tips

You may find it difficult to lower your knees toward the floor. If your knees are incredibly high and your back is rounded, be sure to sit on a high support, even as high as a foot off the floor.

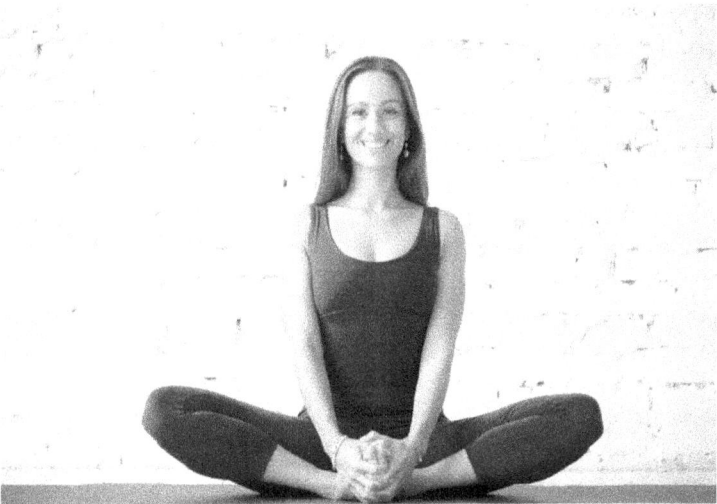

Hero Pose (Virasana)

The Hero Pose is one of the most classical seated yoga postures that stretch the thighs and ankles while improving posture. It is one of the most ancient and traditional postures used for meditation and breathing exercises.

How to Do

Begin in a straight kneeling pose with your hips over your knees and the tops of your feet flat on your mat. Keep your knees together, moving your feet to either side until they are roughly a foot and a half away from each other. You should be extending your feet apart to make space for your bottom to descend to the floor between them, while your feet are separating but the knees are staying together.

Take care that you are not sitting on your feet, but somewhat between them with the tops of your feet on your mat, with your feet pointing straight back, not turning in or out. Lower your shoulders away from your ears, resting your hands in your lap.

Benefits

The Hero Pose strengthens your arches, stretches your thighs, knees, and ankles.

Tips

If at any time you are experiencing pain or extreme discomfort in your knees, raise the sit bones on a block. If you are going through sensation in the tops of the feet or ankles, try tucking a rolled up blanket or a folded towel beneath the feet for added support.

If your knees begin to bend apart, loop a strap around your thighs to keep the legs together and put off overusing the inside muscles of the thighs.

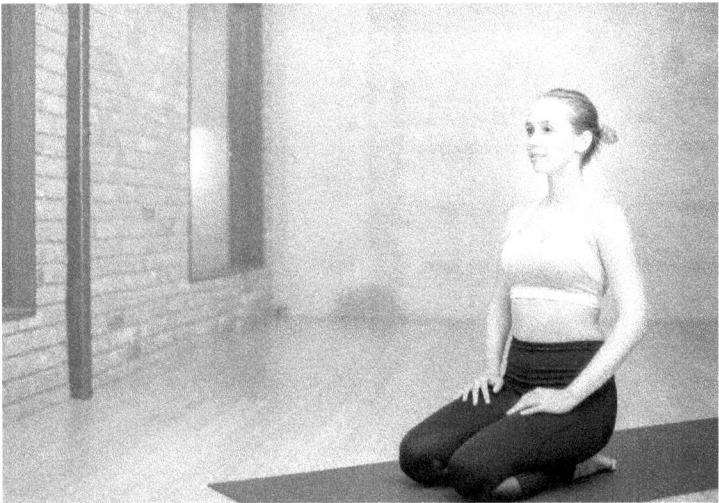

Cow Face Fold Pose (Gomukhasana)

The Cow Face Fold pose is a demanding seated pose. It is a deep hip opener, and is well-known for its complexity to individuals with tight shoulders. It is perceived as being an invigorating, seated deep stretch pose.

How to Do

Begin by sitting on the floor with the feet apart and the knees somewhat bent. Bring the left foot under the right knee and place the heel close to the right hip. Have the toes pointing right. Then bring the right foot close to the left hip, toes pointing to the left. The right knee should now be over the left knee. Keep your weight spread out between the sitting bones. Push the right knee down with both hands to bring them together.

Stretch out your right arm out to the side and turn the shoulder inward so that your palm faces the back and several points downward. Bend the elbow, Palm facing outward; take the right hand behind the back. Stretch the left arm up, turn your arm from the shoulder so that your thumb points backward, and then bend the elbow to grasp the hands behind the back. Move the left elbow back and more to the spine line behind your head and raise the chest.

Stay in this pose about one minute, and then release your hands, legs and then copy on the other side.

Benefits

This pose offers a deep stretch for your armpits, chest, shoulders, thighs, hips, and ankles. It develops your posture by opening the low spine.

Tip

Beginners have a tough time having both sitting bones to support on the floor. Use a bolster or a folded blanket to lift the sitting bones off the floor and support them.

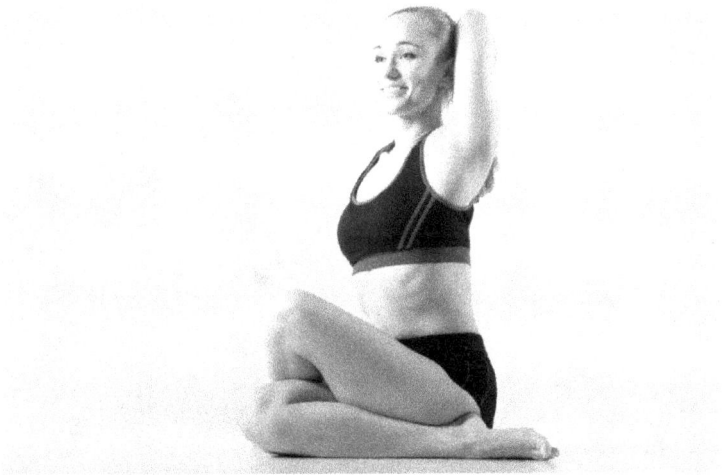

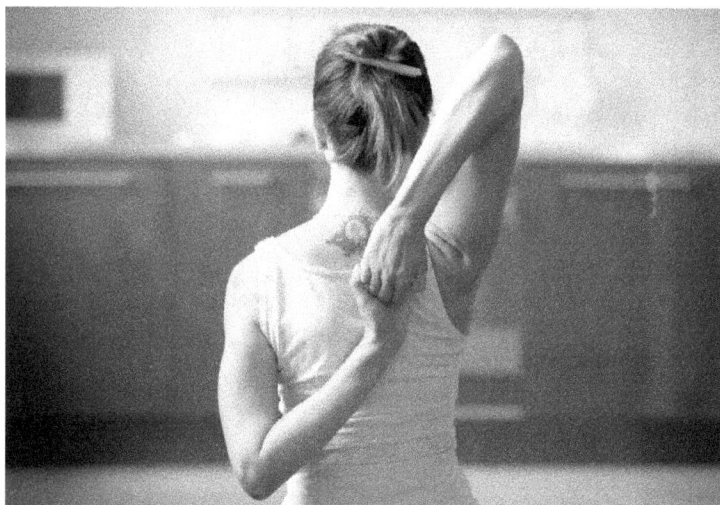

Seated Forward Fold Pose (Paschimottanasana)

The Seated Forward Fold is a calming yoga pose that aids to relieve stress. This pose is frequently performed later in a series, when the body is warm.

How to Do

From the Staff Pose, inhale the arms up over the head and lift and lengthen up through the fingers and crown of the head. Exhale and bend at the hips, slowly drop your torso towards your legs. Reach the hands to the toes, feet or ankles.

To deepen the stretch, use the arms to gently pull the head and torso closer to the legs. Press out through the heels and gently draw the toes towards you. Breathe and hold for five to ten breaths. To release from this pose slowly roll up the spine back into Staff pose. Inhale the arms back over your head as you lift the torso back into the Staff pose.

Benefits

The Seated Forward Fold delivers a deep stretch for the whole back side of your body from the heels to the neck. The Forward Fold soothes your nervous system and emotions.

Tips

By no means should force yourself into a forward bend, particularly when sitting on the floor. Extend forward, when you feel the area between your pubis and navel shortening, you should stop, lift up a little, and lengthen again. Frequently, because of the tightness in the backs of your legs, a beginner's forward bend doesn't go very far forward and may possibly look more like sitting up straight.

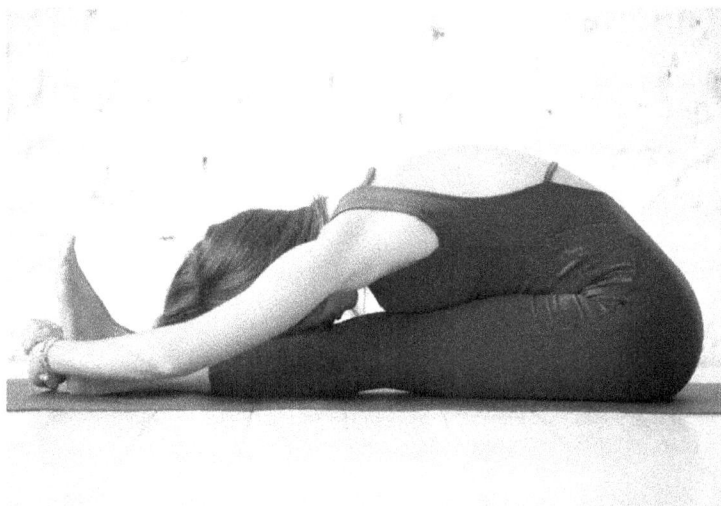

Seated Wide Angle Forward Fold Pose (Upavistha Konasana)

The Seated Wide Angle Forward Fold Pose is a seated yoga pose that deeply elongates your legs and spine, at the same time as calming your mind and releasing stress. It is commonly practiced just before the close of a yoga class, while your body is warm, to get ready your body for even deeper forward bends.

How to Do

Beginning from the Staff Pose, open your legs out as wide as it is comfortable for you. Keep your thighs engaged and your feet arched.

Make sure that your toes are pointing perpendicular to the ceiling as that is the best position for your hips and knees. Don't allow your feet to droop inward or open outward. Press your legs down into the floor.

Breathe in and position down by way of your bottom. Breathe out and forward bend by moving your pelvis forward. Maintain this repetition on each inhale and exhale to deepen the pose.

Let your arms come straight out in front of you and keep your stare softy at the floor to prevent turning your neck.

Benefits

Stimulates your abdominal organs, strengthens the back, stretches your inner thighs and hamstrings and soothes your nervous system.

Tips

Seated Wide Angle Forward Fold Pose is a challenging forward bend for many beginners. If you have trouble bending even a fraction forward, it's okay to bend your knees to some extent. You may possibly even support your knees on rolled blankets or supports; just remember, as you start into the forward bend, it's still essential to keep your kneecaps pointing upwards.

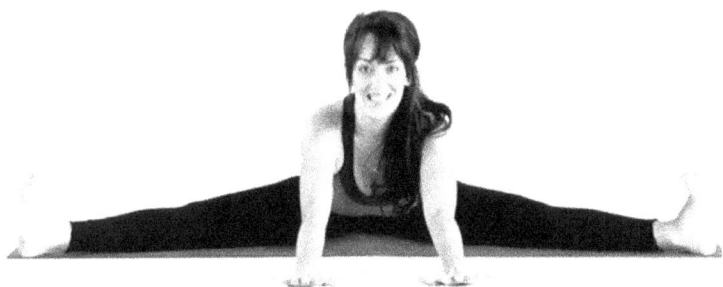

Downward Facing Dog Pose (Adho Mukha Svanasana)

Downward Facing Dog Pose is one of the traditional Sun Salutation sequences poses. It's also an excellent yoga asana all on its own.

How to Do

Begin with your hands and knees in a tabletop position. Make sure your shoulders are aligned above your wrists and your hips are aligned above your knees. Come to a flat back by lengthening the spine. Place your head and neck in a non-aligned position, staring down in the direction of the floor.

Breathe out and raise your knees away from the floor. At the start, keep your knees slightly bent and your heels lifted away from the floor. Lengthen your tailbone positioned from the back of your pelvis and press it slightly toward the pubis. Alongside this tension, raise the resting bones in the direction of the ceiling, and from your inner ankles pull the inner legs up into the groin.

Followed by letting your breath out, push your top thighs back and extend your heels against or down toward the floor. Making sure that you do not lock them, straighten your knees and steady your outer thighs, rolling the upper thighs inward slightly, narrowing the front of the pelvis.

Firming the outer arms, press the bottoms of your index fingers assertively into the floor. From these two points, lift alongside the inside of your arms from the wrists to the tops of the shoulders. Firm your shoulder blades against your back then widen them and draw them toward the tailbone. Keep your head between your upper arms; not allowing it to simply hang.

Continue in this pose somewhere between one to three minutes. Afterward, bend your knees to the floor with a breath and repose in the Child's Pose.

Benefits

Downward Facing Dog pose can help decrease back pain through strengthening the whole back and shoulder girdle. It aids in stronger hands, wrists, the Achilles tendon, low-back, hamstrings, and calves, as well as increasing the full-body circulation. Elongates your shoulders and shoulder blade area. Decrease in tension and headaches by elongating the cervical spine and neck and relaxing the head. It can also lessen anxiety and expand your respiration

Tips

You can alleviate the burden on your wrists by employing a block beneath your palms or you can be capable of completing the pose upon your elbows. By lifting your hands on blocks or the seat of a chair, you can help to release and open your shoulders.

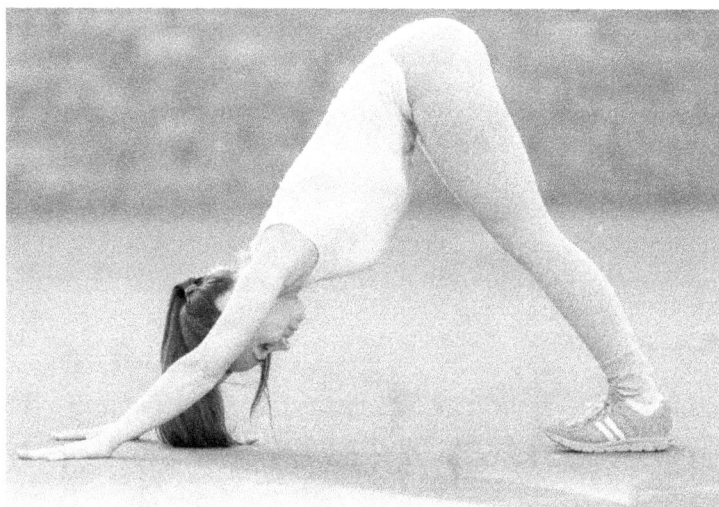

Upward Facing Dog Pose (Urdhva Mukha Svanasana)

Upward Facing Dog Pose is one of the most commonly known, as well as Downward Dog Pose, and recognized yoga pose due to its many benefits and healing uses. Similar to the Cobra Pose, it is thought of as one of the simplest of the back-bending poses and is implemented during the traditional Sun Salutation sequence.

How to Do

Lie face down on the floor. Stretch your legs back, with the tops of your feet on the floor. Bend your elbows and stretch your palms on the floor at the side of your waist so that your forearms are somewhat erect to the floor.

Breathe in and press your inner hands firmly into the floor and somewhat back, similar to trying to push yourself forward along the floor. Then at the same time, straighten your arms and lift your torso up and your legs a few inches off the floor on an intake breath. Keep the thighs firm and somewhat turned inward, the arms firm and turned out so the elbow creases face forward.

Press your tailbone toward your pubis and lift pubis toward your navel. Contract the hip positions. Stiffen but do not totally harden the buttocks.

Steady your shoulder blades against the back and puff the side ribs forward. Lift through the top of the sternum but make an effort not to push the front ribs forward. It will prompt the lower back to tighten. You will at that point look forward or you can angle your head towards the back slightly, remembering to take care not to constrict the back of your neck and the tightening of your throat.

Even though Upward Facing Dog Pose is one position used in the traditional Sun Salutation sequence, you can correspondingly practice this pose independently, maintaining the pose fifteen to thirty seconds, inhaling slowly. Release back to the floor or lift into the Downward Facing Dog pose along with an exhalation.

Benefits

Upward Facing Dog helps open the chest and strengthens the whole body and aligns the spine and invigorates nervous system and the kidneys.

Tips

Performing Upward Facing Dog will elongate and strengthen your whole body. You can use it as a backbend by itself, or as a transition for even deeper backbends.

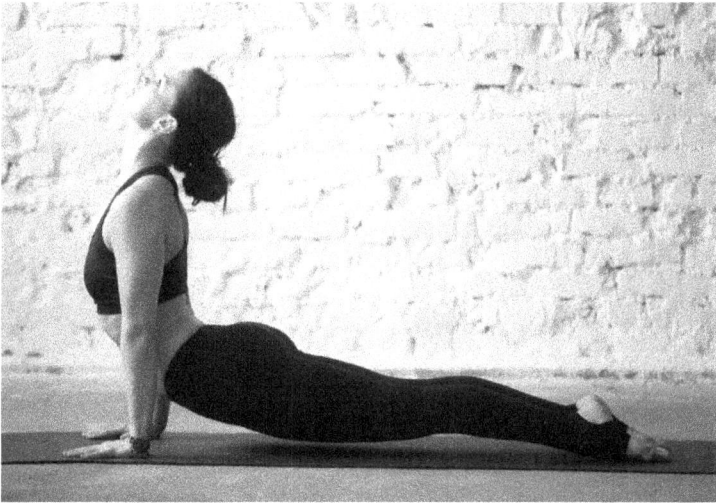

Legs up The Wall Pose (Viparita Karani)

The Legs up the Wall Pose is an upturn pose where you lie on the floor against a wall and position your legs together vertically against the wall.

How to Do

If you are performing the assisted version, place a firm pillow or cushion on the floor against the wall.

Start off the pose by sitting with your right side against the wall. Your lower back should rest against the bolster if you're using one. Slightly turn your body to the right and bring your legs up onto the wall. On the other hand, if you are using a pillow, shift your lower back onto it before bringing your legs up the wall. Use your hands for balance as you transfer your weight.

Drop your back to the floor and lie down. Relax your shoulders and head on the floor. Transfer your weight from side-to-side and move your buttocks close to the wall. Allow your arms to rest open at your sides with your palms facing up. If you're using a pillow, your lower back should at this time be totally held by it.

Allow the part of your bone that connects in the hip socket (the top of your thigh bones) to release and relax, dropping in the direction of the back of your pelvis.

Close your eyes and hold for five to ten minutes, as you breathe with mindfulness.

To release, slowly boost yourself away from the wall and slide your legs down to the left side. Use your hands to help press yourself back up into a seated position.

Benefits

This pose reduces fatigue, cramping in the legs and feet and stretches the back of the legs. It can be an excellent pose for alleviating swollen ankles and calves triggered by long periods of standing pregnancy, and travel. It furthermore elongates the front of the upper body as well as the back of the neck and can be helpful for relieving mild backaches.

Tips

Use your breath to ground the tops of your thighs bones into the wall, which assists in the release of your abdomen, spine, and groins. Imagine in the pose, which each inhalation is falling through your upper body and pushing the tops of your thigh bones closer to the wall. Next with each exhale, hold your thighs to the wall and let your upper body extend over the bolster away from the wall and onto the floor.

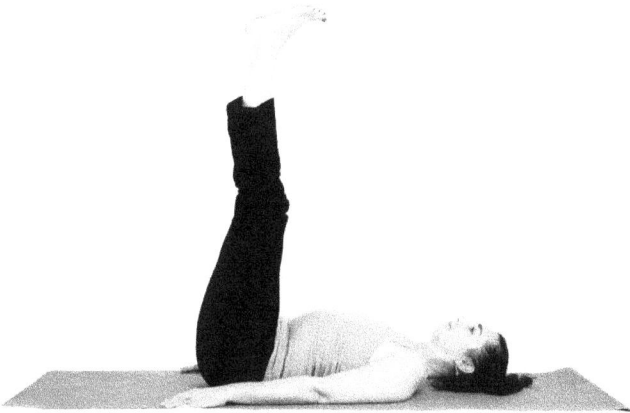

Child's Pose (Balasana)

The Child's Pose is a popular beginner's yoga posture. It is generally utilized as a resting position in among more difficult poses throughout a yoga practice.

How to Do

Come to all fours (Table Pose) exhale and lower your hips to your heels and forehead to the floor. Kneeling on the floor, bring your big toes together and sit on your heels, then separate your knees about as far as your hips.

Your arms can be above your head with your palms on the floor. Your palms can be flat or fisted with them stacked under your forehead, or your arms can be at the sides of your body with your palms up.

The Child's Pose is a resting pose. Remain in this position anywhere from thirty seconds to a few minutes. Beginners can also use this pose to get a feel of a deep forward bend. To come up, first stretch your front torso, followed by an inhalation lift from your tailbone as it pushes down and into your pelvis.

Benefits

The Child's Pose aids to stretch your hips, thighs, and ankles at the same time it reduces stress and fatigue. It gradually relaxes the muscles on the front of your body while softly and reflexively elongates the muscles of the back of your torso.

As it centers, calm, and soothes your brain, the Child's Pose is said to be a beneficial posture for alleviating stress. When done with your head and torso braced, it can as well help relieve back and neck pain.

The Child's Pose soothes the body, mind, and spirit while stimulating your third eye. Gently stretching the lower back, the Child's Pose massages and tones your abdominal organs, and encourages digestion and elimination.

Tips

Before you relax completely, press your palms into the ground with your arms straight and elbows lifted. Push your hips firmly back toward your heels. Breathe deeply into your whole back, for an extra release in your back. Make use of this pose to rest in the middle of more challenging poses.

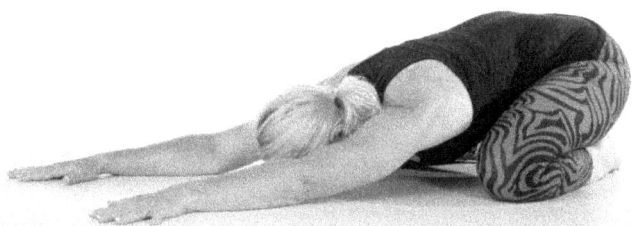

Constructing a Yoga Sequence

Here are a few points to keep in mind how to construct a yoga sequence. You are not at a studio, paying to be there. You do not have to exercise for over an hour. Begin with 5-10 minutes. Notice how you feel by the end of this time. If you feel as if you can do more, go ahead. If no, end your routine there.

Start with 5-10 minutes. By the conclusion of that time, notice how you feel. Do you desire to resume? If yes, continue for an extra five minutes and then check in with yourself once more. If not, close your workout.

The same as any physical journey, a yoga sequence has three clear parts.

Your opening or warm-up sequence

You don't want to jump into the main event tight and cold. This is where you move through and loosening up your major muscle groups as well as body parts

Your main sequence

Once you've warmed up, it's time for your main sequence. This component of your sequence is influenced by the goal of your routine. If it's an asymmetrical pose, keep in mind to do both sides and devote about the same time on each side.

The closing or cool down sequence

Now you've completed the principal portion of your yoga practice, it's time to cool down.

About The Author

Monique Joiner Siedlak is a writer, witch, and warrior on a mission to awaken people to their greatest potential through the power of storytelling infused with mysticism, modern paganism, and new age spirituality. At the young age of 12, she began rigorously studying the fascinating philosophy of Wicca. By the time she was 20, she was self-initiated into the craft, and hasn't looked back ever since. To this day, she has authored over 35 books pertaining to the magick and mysteries of life. Her most recent publication is book one of an Urban Paranormal series entitled "Jaeger Chronicles."

Originally from Long Island, New York, Monique is now a proud inhabitant of Northeast Florida; however, she considers herself to be a citizen of Mother Earth. When she doesn't have a book or pen in hand, she loves exploring new places and learning new things. And being the nature lover that she is, she considers herself to be an avid animal advocate.

To find out more about Monique Joiner Siedlak artistically, spiritually, and personally, feel free to visit her **official website**.

Other Books by Monique Joiner Siedlak

Mojo's Wiccan Series

Wiccan Basics

Candle Magick

Wiccan Spells

Love Spells

Abundance Spells

Hoodoo

Herb Magick

Seven African Powers: The Orishas

Moon Magick

Cooking for the Orishas

Creating Your Own Spells

Body Mind and Soul Series

Creative Visualization

Astral Projection for Beginners

Meditation for Beginners

Reiki for Beginners

Thorne Witch Series

The Phoenix

Beautiful You Series

Creating Your Own Body Butter

Creating Your Own Body Scrub

Creating Your Own Body Spray

Mojo's Self-Improvement Series

Manifesting With the Law of Attraction

Stress Management

Jaeger Chronicles

Glen Cove

Connect With Me!

I really appreciate you reading my book! Please leave a review and let me know your thoughts. Here are the social media locations you can find me at:

Like my Facebook Page: www.facebook.com/mojosiedlak

Follow me on Twitter: www.twitter.com/mojosiedlak

Follow me on Instagram: www.instagram.com/mojosiedlak

Follow me on Bookbub: http://bit.ly/2KEMkqt

Sign up to my Email List at www.mojosiedlak.com and receive a free book!

If you enjoyed this book or found it useful I'd be very grateful if you'd post a short review at your retailer. Your support really does make a difference and I read all the reviews personally so I can get your feedback and make this as well as the next book even better.